94 Juice and Meal Recipes for People Who Have Had a Loss of Appetite:

Increase Hunger and Improve Appetite by Eating Delicious and Filling Foods

By

Joe Correa CSN

COPYRIGHT

This publication is designed to provide accurate and authoritative information in regard to the subject matter covered. It is sold with the understanding that neither the author nor the publisher is engaged in rendering medical advice. If medical advice or assistance is needed, consult with a doctor. This book is considered a guide and should not be used in any way detrimental to your health. Consult with a physician before starting this nutritional plan to make sure it's right for you.

ACKNOWLEDGEMENTS

This book is dedicated to my friends and family that have had mild or serious illnesses so that you may find a solution and make the necessary changes in your life.

94 Juice and Meal Recipes for People Who Have Had a Loss of Appetite:

Increase Hunger and Improve Appetite by Eating Delicious and Filling Foods

By

Joe Correa CSN

CONTENTS

Copyright

Acknowledgements

About The Author

Introduction

94 Juice and Meal Recipes for People Who Have Had a Loss of Appetite: Increase Hunger and Improve Appetite by Eating Delicious and Filling Foods

Additional Titles from This Author

ABOUT THE AUTHOR

After years of Research, I honestly believe in the positive effects that proper nutrition can have over the body and mind. My knowledge and experience has helped me live healthier throughout the years and which I have shared with family and friends. The more you know about eating and drinking healthier, the sooner you will want to change your life and eating habits.

Nutrition is a key part in the process of being healthy and living longer so get started today. The first step is the most important and the most significant.

INTRODUCTION

94 Juice and Meal Recipes for People Who Have Had a Loss of Appetite: Increase Hunger and Improve Appetite by Eating Delicious and Filling Foods

By Joe Correa CSN

From my own experience, I have created these delicious recipes that helped me boost my own appetite and have a balanced diet full of nutrients.

The key to healing this condition and regaining a healthy appetite lies in a healthy diet. The right amount of nutrients are crucial in getting your body back in balance. Furthermore, you will have to learn what and how to eat, you will have to time your meals to get your metabolism back in track.

Having a schedule for eating the right foods is the important in order to increase appetite. It doesn't mean you have to eat tons of food every meal. On the contrary, it means eating smaller portions of food 5-6 times per day with a wide range of healthy snacks included into your daily diet.

The best possible way to get the right nutrients out of the food you're eating is to consume freshly prepared meals and juices. Lots of fruits and vegetables loaded with vitamins, minerals, and fiber, are an ideal solution to cleaning your body and improving your digestive tract.

This book offers a collection of healthy and delicious meal and juice recipes that will increase your appetite in no time. Plus, they are loaded with iron-rich foods that will help you get rid of anemia within just a few days.

Get started today and see the results.

94 JUICE AND MEAL RECIPES FOR PEOPLE WHO HAVE HAD A LOSS OF APPETITE

Meals

1.   Cheddar Cheese Casserole

Ingredients:

4 free range eggs

1 cup of cheddar cheese, crumbled

1 bell pepper, chopped

1 medium-sized onion, sliced

2 large potatoes, shredded

½ tsp of salt

½ tsp of black pepper, ground

1 tbsp of olive oil

1 tsp of parsley

Preparation:

Preheat the oven to 370°F.

Heat up the oil over in a large frying skillet over a medium-high temperature. Add the onion and stir-fry for 1 minute.

Now, add potatoes and pepper. Cook for about 5 minutes, or until potatoes nicely crisp. Stir constantly. Remove from the heat and transfer to a baking dish.

Pour the eggs over and add crumbled cheese. Reduce the temperature to low and bake for 20 minutes or until doneness. Remove from the oven and sprinkle with fresh parsley. Set aside to cool.

Serve.

Nutrition information per serving: Kcal: 292, Protein: 17.5g, Carbs: 5.8g, Fats: 1.4g

2.   Orange Cranberry Smoothie

Ingredients:

¼ cup of orange juice

¼ cup of cranberries

½ cup of Greek yogurt

¼ cup of skim milk

1 tbsp of chia seeds

1 tsp of fresh mint, minced

Preparation:

Combine all in a blender. Blend until smooth and transfer to a large serving glasses. Top with fresh mint and refrigerate at least 1 hour before serving.

Enjoy!

Nutrition information per serving: Kcal: 326, Protein: 13.1g, Carbs: 32.4g, Fats: 10.6g

3.　　Cornflour Chicken Breasts

Ingredients:

2 chicken breasts, boneless, skinless, and thinly sliced

2 cups of cornflour

2 medium-sized tomatoes, chopped

3 garlic cloves, minced

1 large egg

1 tsp of vegetable seasoning mix

½ tsp of black pepper, ground

½ tsp of Cayenne pepper, ground

1 tbsp of vegetable oil

1 tbsp of sour cream

Preparation:

Preheat the oven to 400°F.

Combine cornflour, tomato, garlic, cayenne pepper and vegetable seasoning mix in a food processor. Blend until smooth mixture. Set aside.

Whisk the egg in a bowl. Dip the meat in egg, and place to large greased baking sheet. Pour the blended mixture over and coat well with a spoon.

Bake for 20 minutes, or until chicken fork-tender. Remove from the heat and set aside to cool. Top with sour cream for some extra taste.

Nutrition information per serving: Kcal: 244, Protein: 25.3g, Carbs: 22.8g, Fats: 5.7g

4.   Peach & Blueberries Parfait

Ingredients:

1 large peach, chopped

½ cup of sour cream

1 cup of blueberries

1 tbsp of honey

1 tbsp of almonds, finely chopped

Preparation:

Layer the ingredients as listed. Repeat layers until full glasses.

Drizzle with pomegranate seeds on top.

Refrigerate for 30 minutes before serving.

Nutrition information per serving: Kcal: 310, Protein: 12.4g, Carbs: 43.2g, Fats: 7.7g

5.   Spicy Rice and Broccoli

Ingredients

2 cups of white rice, long-grain

1 lb of broccoli, halved

1 cup of button mushrooms, chopped

1/2 cup of sweet cream

1 cup of cottage cheese, shredded

½ tsp od salt

2 tbsp of olive oil

½ tsp of red pepper flakes

Preparation:

Preheat the oven to 370°F.

Cook the rice using package instructions. Drain and set aside.

Combine mushrooms, sweet cream and a pinch of salt in food processor. Blend until creamy mixture. Set aside.

Gently, place the broccoli in a boiling water and cook for 5 minutes. Remove from the heat and drain well.

Grease a baking sheet with oil. Spread the rice equally over. Now add broccoli and spread over the rice.

Spoon mushroom cream on top. Bake for 40 minutes. remove from the oven and cut into cubes for serving. Drizzle with cheese and red pepper flakes.

Nutrition information per serving: Kcal: 293, Protein: 17.4g, Carbs: 42.7g, Fats: 8.7g

6.   Mexican Turkey Patties

Ingredients:

1 lb of ground turkey

½ cup of apple cider vinegar

¼ tsp of garlic, minced

¼ tsp of cumin, ground

1 tsp od fresh coriander, finely chopped

¼ tsp of chili pepper, ground

1 tbsp of vegetable oil

Preparation:

Combine all ingredients in a large bowl. Stir all well to combine. Using your hands, form the patties.

Heat up the oil in a large frying pan over a medium-high temperature. Gently place the patties using a spatula. Cook for about 10 minutes on each side.

Remove from the heat and drain with paper towels.

Serve with some fresh vegetable salad or yogurt.

You can freeze the mixture and use it later as well.

Nutrition information per serving: Kcal: 104, Protein: 16.8g, Carbs: 41.3g, Fats: 11.7g

7.   Beet & Blueberries Smoothie

Ingredients:

1 medium-sized beet, chopped

¼ cup of blueberries, frozen

¼ cup of vanilla yogurt

1 tsp of lemon juice

1 tsp of lemon zest

1 tbsp of honey, raw

Preparation:

Combine beet, blueberries, vanilla yogurt, honey, and lemon juice in a food processor. Blend until smooth.

Top with lemon zest and blueberries for extra taste. Refrigerate for 1 hour before serving.

Nutrition information per serving: Kcal: 119, Protein: 4.2g, Carbs: 14.5g, Fats: 5.3g

8.   Mozzarella Toast

Ingredients:

2 garlic clove, minced

2 tbsp of olive oil

1 tsp of fresh parsley, finely chopped

3 oz of Mozzarella cheese, sliced

4 bread slices, toasted

Preparation:

Place the bread slices in the toaster and set to light brown. Using a kitchen brush, spread the oil over the bread slices. Make a fine layer of cheese and sprinkle with a pinch of fresh parsley.

You can add tomato slices or lettuce leaf for some extra taste. This is, however, optional.

Nutrition information per serving: Kcal: 142, Protein: 6.3g, Carbs: 6.5g, Fats: 4.3g

9.   Banana Pancakes

Ingredients:

1 large banana, pureed

1 cup of all-purpose flour

2 free-range eggs

1 tbsp of honey

1 tbsp of baking powder

1 cup of skim milk

2 tbsp of vegetable oil

Preparation:

Combine flour, banana, baking powder and honey in a large mixing bowl. Stir well to combine.

In a separate bowl, whisk the eggs, milk and 1 tablespoon of oil. Now, pour this mixture into the flour bowl. Use a hand mixer to make a nice lumpy batter.

Heat up 1 tablespoon of oil in a frying pan over a medium-high temperature.

Now pour about ¼ cup of batter onto the pan and cook until browned, and then flip over with a wide spatula.

Repeat the process until done.

Serve pancakes with honey or some fresh fruits by your choice.

Nutrition information per serving: Kcal: 235, Protein: 7.2g, Carbs: 48.2g, Fats: 5.3g

10.   Eggs & Green Onions Soup

Ingredients:

4 cups of chicken broth

2 large eggs

2 egg whites

1 cup of green onions, chopped

1 garlic clove, minced

1 tsp of salt

½ tsp of black pepper, ground

2 large potatoes, peeled and cut into bite-sized pieces

1 medium-sized carrot, sliced

1 tsp of cornstarch

1 cup of green onions

1 tsp of finely chopped parsley

Preparation:

Pour the vegetable broth into a deep pot over a medium-high temperature. Bring it to a boil and remove from the heat. Set aside.

In a separate pot, combine potatoes and carrot . Add a pinch of salt and bring cook for about 10 minutes, or until potatoes are fork-tender. Remove from the heat and drain well. Transfer to the vegetable broth.

Whisk the eggs and egg whites properly and stir it in the pot. Add remaining spices and cover with a lid. Reduce the temperature to low, and cook for 15 minutes.

Nutrition information per serving: Kcal: 325, Protein: 21.7g, Carbs: 47.2g, Fats: 7.3g

11.   Marinated Trout

Ingredients:

2 lbs of trout, cleaned

2 large potatoes, peeled and cut into wedges

For the marinade:

3 tbsp of olive oil

3 garlic cloves, crushed

1 tbsp of fresh rosemary, finely chopped

1 tsp of white pepper, crushed

1 tsp of dried thyme, ground

1 tsp of salt

3 bay leaves

Preparation:

Combine marinade ingredients in a large baking sheet. Set aside.

Wash and pat dry the fish. Place it into the marinade and coat well. Refrigerate for one hour.

Preheat the oven to 400°F.

Add potato wedges and bake for 25 to 30 minutes, or until fish is fork-tender. Serve with lemon slices.

Nutrition information per serving: Kcal: 279, Protein: 24.6g, Carbs: 56.7g, Fats: 14.8g

12.   Asian Chicken Salad

Ingredients:

1 lb of chicken breasts, pre-cooked, cut into bite-sized pieces

1 cup of spring onions, chopped

1 cup of celery, chopped

½ cup of fresh parsley, finely chopped

1 tsp of fresh coriander, finely chopped

2 cups of Romaine lettuce, chopped

For dressing:

1 tbsp of balsamic vinegar

2 tbsp of orange juice

1 tsp of salt

1 tbsp of vegetable oil

1 tsp of sesame seeds

1 tsp of almond, roughly chopped

¼ tsp of black pepper, ground

Preparation:

Combine all ingredients except chicken, in a large bowl. Stir once and set aside.

Combine all dressing ingredients in a mixing bowl. Stir well and set aside to allow flavors to meld for about 10 minutes.

Drizzle the dressing over the vegetables and top with chicken chops. Sprinkle with pepper for extra taste.

Nutrition information per serving: Kcal: 246, Protein: 24.6g, Carbs: 98.7g, Fats: 10.3g

13.   Sweet Veal Steaks

Ingredients:

1 lb of veal steaks, boneless, thinly sliced

1 orange, peeled and cut into wedges

½ of small lemon, peeled

1 tbsp of yellow mustard

1 tbsp of honey

2 tbsp of balsamic vinegar

½ tsp of salt

½ tsp of black pepper, ground

1 tbsp of basil, finely chopped

Preparation:

Preheat the oven to 400°F.

Combine orange, lemon, mustard, honey, and vinegar in a food processor. Blend until smooth and set aside.

Place the steaks in a large baking sheet. Pour the mixture over and sprinkle with salt and pepper.

Bake for 45 to 50 minutes, or until doneness. Remove from the oven and serve with fresh basil.

Nutrition information per serving: Kcal: 121, Protein: 16.2g, Carbs: 12.3g, Fats: 5.6g

14.   Couscous Tomato Salad

Ingredients:

3 large tomatoes, diced

1 cup of couscous

½ cup of Mozzarella cheese, diced

2 tbsp of fresh spring onions, finely chopped

2 tbsp of olive oil

1 tbsp of lemon juice

1 garlic clove, crushed

¼ tsp of black pepper, ground

1 tsp of fresh basil, finely chopped

1 cup of water

½ tsp of red pepper flakes

Preparation:

Combine tomatoes, cheese, lemon juice, spring onions, olive oil, garlic, salt, and pepper in a mixing bowl. Cover with a lid and refrigerate. Marinate for about 30 minutes to allow flavors to meld.

Pour water into a large frying saucepan and bring it to a boil. Stir in the couscous and remove from the heat immediately. Cover with a lid and set aside for 5 minutes. Stir few times.

Now, combine tomato and cheese mixture with drained couscous in a serving bowl. Stir in the basil and toss well properly.

Sprinkle with red pepper flakes for some extra taste and serve.

Nutrition information per serving: Kcal: 142, Protein: 5.8g, Carbs: 28.4g, Fats: 6.3g

15.   Ziti Beef

Ingredients:

1 lb of beef steak, chopped into bite-sized pieces

2 small onions, sliced

1 large bell pepper, chopped

1 medium-sized zucchini, peeled and cubed

1 cup of tomato sauce

½ tsp of salt

½ tsp of black pepper, crushed

1 tsp of fresh parsley, finely chopped

Preparation:

Preheat the oil in a slow cooker over a medium-high temperature. Add the onions and saute until translucent.

Add meat chops, bell pepper, and zucchini. Sprinkle with some salt and pepper to taste. Stir well to combine.

Seal the lid and reduce the temperature to low. Cook for about 20 minutes, and remove from the heat. Let it stay for 15 minutes, and then open the lid.

Meanwhile, follow the package instructions to cook ziti pasta. Drain well and transfer to a serving plate.

Stir in the beef into the pasta and serve. Top with some fresh parsley.

Serve warm.

Nutrition information per serving: Kcal: 121, Protein: 16.2g, Carbs: 12.3g, Fats: 5.6g

16.   Cabbage Soup

Ingredients:

1 lb of cabbage, shredded

1 cup of celery, chopped

4 medium-sized carrots, sliced

2 garlic cloves, crushed

2 large tomatoes, chopped

1 medium-sized onion, chopped

½ tsp of salt

1 tsp of vegetable seasoning mix

1 cup of vegetable broth

3 cups of water

Preparation:

Combine tomatoes and onions in a blender well until smooth.

Meanwhile, combine all other ingredients in a slow cooker. Add the tomato and onion mixture and stir well.

Cover with lid and cook for 4 hours over a medium-high temperature.

Nutrition information per serving: Kcal: 87, Protein: 2.4g, Carbs: 17.2g, Fats: 6.4g

17.   Red Peppers with Goat's Cheese

Ingredients:

1 cup of Goat's cheese, crumbled

2 large bell peppers, seeded and cut into strips

2 garlic cloves, minced

1 small onion, sliced

1 tbsp of olive oil

1 tbsp of honey

1 tbsp of apple cider vinegar

1 tsp of dried basil, minced

2 lettuce leaves, whole

½ tsp of salt

¼ tsp of black pepper, ground

Preparation:

Preheat the oil in a large frying skillet over a medium-high temperature. Add onions and garlic and stir-fry until translucent. Add peppers and cook for about 10 minutes, or until fork-tender.

Stir in honey, vinegar, basil, salt, and pepper. Cook for 5 more minutes stirring occasionally. Remove from the heat and let it cool for few minutes.

Line lettuce leaves on a serving plate. Transfer the peppers and sauce onto lettuce leaves, and top with cheese.

Nutrition information per serving: Kcal: 165, Protein: 6.5g, Carbs: 4.8g, Fats: 14.3g

18.   Guava Mango Smoothie

Ingredients:

1 medium sized mango, peeled and chopped

1 medium-sized guava, peeled and chopped

½ cup of Greek yogurt

¼ cup of skim milk

1 tbsp of honey

1 tbsp of whipped cream

1 tsp of cocoa, raw

Preparation:

Combine mango, guava, yogurt, milk, and honey in a food processor. Blend until smooth. Transfer to a serving glasses and top with whipped cream. Sprinkle with cocoa for extra taste!

Nutrition information per serving: Kcal: 115, Protein: 4.1g, Carbs: 24.5g, Fats: 1.2g

19.   Spinach & Cheddar Cheese Salad

Ingredients:

5 oz of baby spinach, finely chopped

½ cup of cheddar cheese, crumbled

1 large apple, shredded

For the dressing:

1 tbsp of balsamic vinegar

3 tbsp of extra-virgin olive oil

1 tbsp of Dijon mustard

1 tsp of cumin, ground

1 tsp of vegetable seasoning mix

1 tbsp of water

½ tsp od salt

½ tsp of black pepper, ground

Preparation:

Combine all dressing ingredients in a mixing bowl. Stir well to combine and set aside.

Combine baby spinach and shredded apple in a large serving bowl. Top with cheese. Drizzle with marinade and give a good stir. Set aside for a few minutes to allow flavors to mingle.

Serve immediately.

Nutrition information per serving: Kcal: 420, Protein: 8.2g, Carbs: 15.8g, Fats: 21.6g

20.   Quinoa Chili Stew

Ingredients:

8 oz of button mushrooms, sliced

1 cup of kidney beans, pre-cooked, drained and rinsed

½ lb of chicken breasts, skinless and boneless, cut into bite-sized pieces

1 cup of quinoa, pre-cooked

½ cup of cottage cheese, shredded

1 small chili pepper, chopped

½ tsp of dried oregano, ground

½ tsp of cumin, ground

1 cup of tomato sauce

3 cups of chicken broth, unsalted

½ tsp of fresh coriander, finely chopped

1 cup of water

Preparation:

Place mushrooms and water in a large frying skillet over a medium-low temperature. Cover with a lid and cook for 10 minutes, or until fork-tender. Remove from the heat and set aside.

Combine kidney beans, oregano, cumin, and chili in a food processor. Blend until smooth and transfer to the mushroom skillet. Pour the chicken broth and add chicken chops and tomato sauce.

Add quinoa and coriander. Give it a good stir to combine. Cover with a lid and cook for 20 minutes. Remove from the heat and stir in the cheese. Set aside for few minutes to cool.

Top with fresh coriander and serve warm.

Nutrition information per serving: Kcal: 210, Protein: 17.8g, Carbs: 32.4g, Fats: 5.7g

21.   Raisins and Carrot Salad

Ingredients:

1 cup of raisins, chopped

5 medium sized carrots, sliced

1 cup of spring onions, chopped

¼ cup of almonds, roughly chopped

For the dressing:

2 tbsp of lemon juice

2 tbsp of olive oil

½ tsp of curry powder

1 tbsp of maple syrup

Preparation:

Combine all dressing ingredients in a mixing bowl. Stir all well to combine and set aside.

Now combine all salad ingredients in a medium serving bowl and drizzle with dressing. Serve immediately.

Nutrition information per serving: Kcal: 219, Protein: 4.7g, Carbs: 27.8g, Fats: 3.2g

22.   Salmon Green Omelet

Ingredients:

6 free-range eggs

4 oz of wild smoked salmon, skinless, boneless, and cubed

¼ cup of asparagus, chopped

1 garlic clove, crushed

1 tsp of fresh dill, minced

1 small onion, sliced

1 tsp of lemon juice

1 tbsp of olive oil

2 tbsp of fresh parsley, finely chopped

1 tbsp of skim milk

½ tsp of salt

¼ tsp of black pepper, ground

Preparation:

Beat the eggs in mixing bowl. Add milk, dill, parsley, salt, and pepper. Whisk well to combine and set aside.

Meanwhile, heat up the oil in a large frying skillet over a medium-high temperature. Add garlic and onions. Stir-fry for 5 minutes, or until translucent. Add asparagus and lemon juice. Cook for 4-5 minutes stirring occasionally.

Add the eggs mixture and cook for 3-4 minutes and flip the omelet. Now add salmon chops, and cook for 2 minutes more. Remove from the heat and serve warm.

Nutrition information per serving: Kcal: 169, Protein: 12.5g, Carbs: 5.3g, Fats: 10.3g

23. Oatmeal Smoothie

Ingredients:

½ cup of oatmeal

½ cup of Greek yogurt

1 tbsp of honey

½ cup of fresh strawberries, halved

1 tbsp of quinoa

Preparation:

Combine all ingredients in a blender. Blend until smooth and transfer to a serving glass. Top with quinoa for some extra nutrients!

Refrigerate for 30 minutes before serving.

Nutrition information per serving: Kcal: 212, Protein: 19.8g, Carbs: 33.6g, Fats: 1.8g

24.   Black & White Soup

Ingredients:

5 oz of white beans

5 oz of black beans

2 medium-sized red onions, minced

1 medium-sized carrot, sliced

4 oz of Brussel sprouts, halved

2 garlic cloves, finely chopped

5 cups of chicken broth, (or vegetable broth for vegetarians)

½ tsp of black pepper, ground

½ tsp of sea salt

1 tbsp of vegetable oil

Preparation:

Place beans and lentils in a large pot. Pour enough water to cover all and bring it to a boil over a high temperature. Remove from the heat and let it soak in the water for about 1 hour. Drain well and set aside.

Meanwhile, heat up the oil in a deep pot over a medium-high temperature. Add onions and stir-fry for few minutes, until translucent. Add Brussel sprouts and carrot. Cook for about two minutes, stirring occasionally. Now, pour in 5 cups of chicken broth, and add pre-cooked beans and lentils. Adjust the thickness of the soup with broth. Add a pinch of salt and pepper to taste.

Reduce the temperature to low, and cover with a lid. Cook for about 45 minutes. Remove from the heat and let it cool a little bit.

Sprinkle with some fresh parsley. This is, however, optional.

Nutrition information per serving: Kcal: 179, Protein: 11.3g, Carbs: 31.7g, Fats: 15.4g

25.   Warm Peach and Cranberries Porridge

Ingredients:

½ cup of dried peaches, chopped

½ cup of dried cranberries, chopped

1 tbsp of flaxseeds

¼ cup of skim milk (or coconut milk)

1 tbsp of honey

1 tsp of vanilla extract

1 tsp cocoa, raw

Preparation:

Combine peaches, cranberries, and flaxseeds in a medium pot. Pour water to cover all ingredients. Bring it to a boil and reduce the heat to low. Add milk and cook for 2 minutes more. Remove from the heat and stir in the honey and vanilla.

Transfer to a serving bowl and sprinkle with cocoa for extra taste.

Nutrition information per serving: Kcal: 258, Protein: 2.6g, Carbs: 51.4g, Fats: 10.2g

26.   Portobello Mushroom Burgers

Ingredients:

5oz Portobello mushrooms

¼ cup of extra virgin olive oil

2 garlic cloves, crushed

½ tsp of dried oregano, crushed

1 tbsp of parsley, finely chopped

¼ tsp of sea salt

¼ tsp of freshly ground black pepper

3 tbsp of mayonnaise

2 tbsp of cheddar, grated

1 large onion, finely chopped

Preparation:

In a medium-sized bowl, whisk together olive oil, garlic, oregano, parsley, salt, and pepper. Using a kitchen brush, spread the mixture over each mushroom and set aside for 20 minutes.

In another bowl, combine mayonnaise with cheddar and chopped onion. You can add some more salt to taste, but this is optional. Use the mixture to stuff each mushroom.

Preheat the grill pan over medium-high heat. Place the mushrooms, top side up and cook for about 7 minutes, or until lightly charred.

Nutrition information per serving: Kcal: 204, Protein: 10.5g, Carbs: 12.2g, Fats: 15.7g

27. Chicken Scallopini in a Creamy Sauce

Ingredients:

2 chicken breast halves, boneless and skinless

¼ cup of butter

1 garlic clove, crushed

1 tsp of dry oregano

¼ cup of fresh lime juice

1 cup of button mushrooms, sliced

½ cup of Gorgonzola cheese, chopped

1 cup of sour cream

3 tbsp of Parmesan cheese, grated

½ tsp of salt

½ cup of all-purpose flour

1 tbsp of honey

½ cup of wine

Preparation:

In a small bowl, combine the flour with sour cream, butter,

honey, Parmesan cheese, and Gorgonzola. Add fresh lime juice and beat well with electric mixer, on high.

Season each chicken breast half with salt and oregano. Place in a slow cooker. Add the creamy mixture, wine, mushrooms, and garlic.

Cover the pressure cooker and set on low for 6-7 hours.

Useful tip:

You can replace wine with fresh orange juice for sweet taste.

Nutrition information per serving: Kcal: 273, Protein: 45.3g, Carbs: 9.4g, Fats: 4.8g

28.   Almond and Vanilla Smoothie

Ingredients:

½ cup of coconut milk

2 large eggs

1 tbsp of coconut oil

1 tbsp of almonds, minced

1 tsp of pure vanilla extract, sugar-free

½ cup of water

½ tsp of stevia

Preparation:

Place the ingredients in a blender and pulse to combine. Serve cold.

Nutrition information per serving: Kcal: 498 Protein: 31g, Carbs: 5g , Fats: 40g

29.   Broccoli and Beef Pasta Bake

Ingredients:

14 oz of lean ground beef

17oz of dried pasta

12 oz of broccoli, sliced

½ cup tomato paste

1 tsp dry oregano, ground

½ tsp of salt

¼ cup butter, melted

1 tbsp of olive oil

½ cup of Cheddar cheese, grated

Preparation:

Combine the tomato paste with oregano, and melted butter. Stir well.

Heat up the olive oil over a medium-high heat. Add ground beef, season with some salt, and cook until brown, stirring constantly. Remove from the heat. Place sliced broccoli at the bottom of your slow cooker. Then add dried pasta, ground beef, and tomato paste mixture.

Cover and set on low for 4-6 hours, or until pasta is tender. Remove from the heat and spread the grated Cheddar. Cover again and allow the cheese to melt.

Serve warm.

Serving tip:

Top with sour cream or Greek yogurt.

Nutrition information per serving: Kcal: 327, Protein: 13.6g, Carbs: 42.5g, Fats: 12.5g

30.   Mango porridge

Ingredients:

1 medium-sized mango, chopped

1 medium-sized pineapple, chopped

½ cup of butter

2 tbsp of coconut flakes

2 cups of crackers, crushed

1 tsp of honey

Preparation:

Preheat the oven to 375°F.

Combine crushed crackers, honey, and coconut flakes in a mixing bowl.

Melt butter in a frying pan and stir it in the crackers mixture. Stir all well to combine. Set aside.

Place the mango and pineapple chops into a large baking dish. Spread the crackers mixture over the fruits equally. Place it in the oven and bake for 25 minutes, or until fork-tender. Remove from the oven and let it cool for a while.

Top with ice cream ball.

Nutrition information per serving: Kcal: 251, Protein: 8.4g, Carbs: 42.6g, Fats: 7.3g

31.   Beef Stroganoff

Ingredients:

2 lbs of stew beef

1 oz of butter

2 large onions, finely chopped

1 garlic clove, crushed

1 cup of button mushrooms, sliced

½ cup of Gorgonzola, crumbled

1 ½ cup of sour cream

½ tsp of salt

½ tsp of black pepper, ground

¼ cup of water

3 cups of rice, pre-cooked

Preparation:

Combine the ingredients, except the sour cream, in a slow cooker. Cover and set on low for 8 hours.

If you set the heat on high, you can reduce the cooking time to 5 hours.

When done, stir in sour cream and serve.

Nutrition information per serving: Kcal: 292, Protein: 20.6g, Carbs: 41.2g, Fats: 6.2g

32.   Creamy Cheese Avocado

Ingredients:

1 ripe avocado

1 large tomato, finely chopped

1 large onion, peeled and finely chopped

2 tbsp of extra virgin olive oil

2 tbsp of tomato paste, sugar-free

¼ cup of cheddar cheese, shredded

1 tbsp of fresh lime juice

½ tsp of salt

1 tsp of cayenne pepper

Preparation:

Preheat the oven to 350°F. Line some baking paper over a baking sheet and set aside.

Slice the avocado in half and remove the stone. Using a sharp knife, cut criss-cross patterns to allow the spices to penetrate the avocado flesh.

In a medium-sized skillet, heat up the olive oil over medium-high heat. Stir-fry the onion for 2-3 minutes, or until translucent, and add chopped tomato. Continue to cook until fork tender. Now add tomato paste, fresh lime juice, salt, and cayenne pepper. Give it a final stir and remove from the heat.

Fill each avocado half with this mixture and top with cheddar. Bake for 20 minutes.

Nutrition information per serving: Kcal: 410 Protein: 1.4g, Carbs: 9.4g , Fats: 2.6g

33.   Cherry Spinach Smoothie

Ingredients:

½ cup of cherries, frozen or fresh, pit removed

¼ cup of spinach, chopped

1 medium-sized banana, sliced

½ cup of almond milk

1 tbsp of honey

Preparation:

Place the ingredients in a blender and pulse to combine. Serve with some ice cubes.

Nutrition information per serving: Kcal: 58 Protein: 1.4g, Carbs: 9.4g , Fats: 2.6g

34. Cauliflower Macaroni with Italian Garlic Sauce

Ingredients:

6 cups of cauliflower florets

3 large ripe tomatoes

3 tbsp of extra virgin olive oil

2 garlic cloves, crushed

½ tsp of dry oregano

¼ tsp of salt

¼ cup of fresh lime juice

½ cup of coconut flour

1 cup of vegetable broth

Preparation:

Preheat the oven to 350 degrees.

Place cauliflower in a deep pot and add enough water to cover. Boil until done. Remove from the heat and drain. Set aside.

Whisk together vegetable broth with coconut flour. Set aside.

Peel and roughly chop the tomatoes. Make sure you keep all the liquid.

Heat up the olive oil over a medium temperature. Add the garlic and stir-fry for several minutes. Now add tomatoes, oregano, and salt. Reduce the heat to low and cook until the tomatoes have softened. Add lime juice and cook for 10 more minutes stirring constantly. Turn off the heat, add cauliflower and cover.

Let it stand for 10 minutes and transfer to a lightly greased baking sheet. Evenly pour over the vegetable broth.

Bake for 15-20 minutes or until you get a nice color on top.

Nutrition information per serving: Kcal: 293, Protein: 12.5g, Carbs: 9g, Fats: 3.99g

35.   Choco-Coco Smoothie

Ingredients:

1 large egg

1 tbsp of coconut oil

1 tsp of chia seeds

¼ cup coconut milk

½ cup of water

1 tsp of stevia

1 tbsp of raw cocoa, sugar-free

½ tsp of vanilla extract, sugar-free

Preparation:

Place the ingredients in a blender and pulse to combine. Serve cold.

Nutrition information per serving: Kcal: 293, Protein: 12.5g, Carbs: 9g, Fats: 3.99g

36. Hot Vege Pizza Stuffed Peppers

Ingredients:

3 large green bell peppers

2 large tomatoes, roughly chopped

2 tbsp of tomato pizza sauce, sugar-free

1 tsp of dried oregano

½ tsp of thyme

4oz Mozzarella cheese, sliced

3 tbsp of parmesan cheese

1 tbsp parsley, finely chopped

4 tbsp of extra virgin olive oil

½ tsp of salt

¼ tsp of black pepper, freshly ground

Preparation:

Preheat the oven to 350 degrees. Line some baking paper over a baking sheet and set aside.

Using a sharp knife, cut the peppers in half and remove the seeds. Grease each paper inside with some olive oil. Set aside.

In a medium-sized bowl, combine mozzarella with tomatoes, pizza tomato sauce, thyme, oregano, parsley, and two tablespoons of olive oil. Stir well and use the mixture to stuff each pepper half. Add some salt and pepper and top with parmesan.

Bake for 20 minutes.

Nutrition information per serving: Kcal: 205, Protein: 11g, Carbs: 5g, Fats: 12g

Juices

1.   Apple Avocado Juice

Ingredients:

1 large Golden Delicious apple, cored

1 cup of avocado, cubed

1 cup of collard greens, chopped

1 cup of fresh mint, chopped

1 oz of milk

Preparation:

Peel the avocado and cut into half. Remove the pit and cut into small cubes. Fill the measuring cup and reserve the rest in the refrigerator.

Wash the apple and cut in half. Remove the core and cut into bite-sized pieces. Set aside.

Combine collard greens and mint in a colander. Wash thoroughly under cold running water and slightly drain. Chop all into small pieces and set aside.

Now, combine avocado, collard greens, mint, and apple in a juicer. Process until well juiced. Transfer to a serving glass and stir in the milk.

Serve immediately.

Nutrition information per serving: Kcal: 324, Protein: 6.6g, Carbs: 48.8g, Fats: 23.2g

2.   Artichoke Pepper Juice

Ingredients:

1 cup of artichoke, chopped

1 large yellow bell pepper, chopped

1 cup of Brussels sprouts, halved

1 oz of water

Preparation:

Trim off the outer leaves of the artichoke. Wash it and cut into small pieces. Fill the measuring cup and reserve the rest in the refrigerator.

Wash the bell pepper and cut lengthwise in half. Remove the seeds and the top stem. Cut into small pieces and set aside.

Wash the Brussels sprouts and trim off the wilted layers. Cut each in half and fill the measuring cup. Set aside.

Now, combine artichoke, pepper, and Brussels sprouts in a juicer and process until juiced. Transfer to a serving glass and stir in the water.

Serve immediately.

Nutrition information per serving: Kcal: 106, Protein: 9.6g, Carbs: 30.9g, Fats: 1.3g

3.   Banana Ginger Juice

Ingredients:

1 large banana, chopped

2 tsp of fresh ginger, grated

1 cup of collard greens, chopped

1 small Granny Smith's apple, cored

1 cup of Brussels sprouts, halved

1 oz of coconut water

Preparation:

Peel the banana and cut into small chunks. Set aside.

Peel and cut one small ginger knob. Grind it and reserve the rest.

Wash the apple and cut in half. Remove the core and cut into bite-sized pieces. Set aside.

Wash the collard greens thoroughly under cold running water and slightly drain. Chop into small pieces and set aside.

Wash the Brussels sprouts and remove the outer wilted layers. Cut each in half and set aside.

Now, combine kale, banana, apple, and Brussels sprouts in a juicer and process until juiced. Transfer to a serving glass and stir in the coconut water and ginger. Add more ginger if you like it spicier.

Add some ice and serve immediately.

Nutrition information per serving: Kcal: 223, Protein: 7.9g, Carbs: 64.4g, Fats: 1.6g

4. Guava Pineapple Juice

Ingredients:

1 cup avocado, chopped

1 cup of pineapple, chunked

1 whole cucumber, sliced

1 cup of fresh mint, torn

1 oz of water

Preparation:

Peel the avocado and cut in half. Remove the pit and cut into chunks. Reserve the rest in the refrigerator.

Cut the top of the pineapple and peel it using a sharp paring knife. Peel it and cut into small pieces. Set aside.

Wash the cucumber and cut into thin slices. Fill the measuring cup and reserve the rest in the refrigerator.

Wash the mint and slightly drain. Torn with hands and set aside.

Now, combine guava, pineapple, cucumber, and mint in a juicer and process until juiced. Transfer to a serving glass and stir in the water.

Refrigerate for 10 minutes before serving.

Nutrition information per serving: Kcal: 317, Protein: 6.7g, Carbs: 48.7g, Fats: 22.1g

5.   Apple Cantaloupe Juice

Ingredients:

1 small Granny Smith's apple, cored

1 large wedge of cantaloupe, chopped

1 cup of fresh mint, chopped

1 cup of mustard greens, chopped

1 oz of milk

Preparation:

Wash the apple and cut lengthwise in half. Remove the core and cut into bite-sized pieces. Set aside.

Cut the cantaloupe in half. Cut one large wedge and peel it. Cut into small pieces and set aside. Wrap the rest of the melon in a plastic foil and refrigerate for later.

Combine mint and mustard greens in a colander and wash thoroughly. Slightly drain and chop into small pieces. Set aside.

Now, combine apple, cantaloupe, mint, and mustard greens in a juicer and process until juiced.

Transfer to a serving glass and stir in the water. Refrigerate for 5 minutes before serving.

Nutrition information per serving: Kcal: 152, Protein: 5.6g, Carbs: 41.7g, Fats: 1.3g

6.   Cinnamon Banana Juice

Ingredients:

1 small banana, chunked

¼ tsp of cinnamon, ground

1 cup of watermelon, cubed

1 cup of cantaloupe, diced

1 oz milk

Preparation:

Peel the banana and cut into chunks. Set aside.

Cut the watermelon lengthwise in half. For one cup, cut one large wedge. Peel and chop into small cubes. Remove the seeds and fill the measuring cup. Reserve the rest in the refrigerator.

Cut the cantaloupe in half and scoop out the seeds. Cut and peel two medium wedges. Fill the measuring cup and reserve the rest for later.

Now, combine banana, watermelon, cantaloupe, and cinnamon in a juicer and process until juiced. Transfer to a serving glass and refrigerate for 10 minutes before serving.

Enjoy!

Nutrition information per serving: Kcal: 186, Protein: 4.3g, Carbs: 48.3g, Fats: 1.3g

7.   Cucumber Yam Juice

Ingredients:

1 cup of sweet potatoes, cubed

1 medium-sized artichoke,chopped

1 cup of cucumber, sliced

1 cup of green cabbage, chopped

Preparation:

Wash the cucumber and cut into thin slices. fill the measuring cup and reserve the rest for later.

Peel the sweet potato and cut into small cubes. Place in a pot of boiling water and cook for 10 minutes. When done, drain and set aside.

Using a sharp paring knife, peel the artichoke and cut into bite-sized pieces. Set aside.

Wash the cabbage thoroughly under cold running water and torn with hands. Set aside.

Now, combine cucumber, sweet potatoes, artichoke, and cabbage in a juicer and process until juiced. Transfer to a serving glass and refrigerate for 5 minutes before serving.

Enjoy!

Nutrition information per serving: Kcal: 150, Protein: 7.7g, Carbs: 47.3g, Fats: 0.4g

8.   Pear Banana Juice

Ingredients:

1 small pear, cored and chopped

1 medium-sized banana, peeled and chunked

1 small Red Delicious apple, cored

1 small ginger knob, peeled and sliced

1 cup of fresh spinach, chopped

Preparation:

Wash the pear and remove the core. Cut into small pieces and set aside.

Peel the banana and cut into small chunks. Set aside.

Wash the apple and cut in half. Remove the core and cut into bite-sized pieces. Set aside.

Peel the ginger knob and chop into small pieces. Set aside.

Wash the spinach thoroughly under cold running water. Slightly drain and chop into small pieces. Set aside.

Now, combine pear, banana, apple, ginger, and spinach in

a juicer and process until juiced. Transfer to a serving glass and refrigerate for 5 minutes before serving.

Enjoy!

Nutrition information per serving: Kcal: 247, Protein: 1.7g, Carbs: 73.9g, Fats: 1.7g

9.   Coconut Carrot Juice

Ingredients:

1 oz of coconut water

1 large carrot, sliced

1 small Golden Delicious apple, cored and chopped

1 cup of mango, chunked

Preparation:

Wash and peel the carrot. Cut into bite-sized pieces and set aside.

Wash the apple and cut in half. Remove the core and cut into bite-sized pieces. Set aside.

Peel the mango and cut into chunks. Fill the measuring cup and reserve the rest for later.

Now, combine carrot, apple, and mango in a juicer and process until juiced. Transfer to a serving glass and stir in the coconut water. Add some crushed ice and serve immediately.

Enjoy!

Nutrition information per serving: Kcal: 179, Protein: 2.6g, Carbs: 51.2g, Fats:1.1g

10.   Banana Melon Juice

Ingredients:

1 medium-sized banana, peeled and chunked

1 cup of watermelon, diced

1 cup of celery, chopped

1 oz of water

Preparation:

Peel the banana and cut into small chunks. Set aside.

Cut the watermelon in half. For one cup, you'll need one large wedge. Peel and dice into small pieces. Remove the pits and fill the measuring cup. Wrap the rest of the melon in a plastic foil and refrigerate for later.

Wash the celery and cut into bite-sized pieces. Fill the measuring cup and reserve the rest for later.

Now, combine banana, watermelon, and celery in a juicer and process until juiced. Transfer to a serving glass and stir in the water.

Add some ice and serve immediately.

Enjoy!

Nutrition information per serving: Kcal: 147, Protein: 2.9g, Carbs: 41.4g, Fats: 0.8g

11.   Pineapple Apricot Juice

Ingredients:

1 cup of pineapple, chunked

5 large apricots, pitted and chopped

¼ tsp of cinnamon, ground

1 small wedge of cantaloupe

Preparation:

Cut the top of the pineapple and peel it using a sharp paring knife. Peel it all and cut into small pieces. Fill the measuring cup and set aside.

Wash apricots and cut in half. Remove the pits and cut into bite-sized pieces. Set aside.

Cut the cantaloupe in half and scoop out the seeds. Cut and peel two medium wedges. Fill the measuring cup and reserve the rest for later.

Now, combine pineapple, apricots, and cantaloupe, in a juicer and process until juiced. Transfer to a serving glass and stir in the cinnamon.

Refrigerate for 5 minutes before serving.

Nutrition information per serving: Kcal: 237, Protein: 5.4g, Carbs: 69.1g, Fats: 5.4g

12.   Spicy Apple Cucumber Juice

Ingredients:

1 small Red Delicious apple, chopped

1 cup of cucumber, sliced

1 cup of green beans, chopped

2 cups of turnip greens, chopped

½ tsp ginger, ground

Preparation:

Wash the apple and cut in half. Remove the core and cut into bite-sized pieces. Set aside.

Wash the cucumber and cut into thin slices. Fill the measuring cup and reserve the rest in the refrigerator. Set aside.

Rinse the beans and place in a pot of boiling water. Cook for 10 minutes and remove from the heat. Drain and chop into small pieces.

Wash the turnip greens thoroughly under cold running water. Chop into small pieces and set aside.

Peel the ginger and cut into small pieces. Set aside.

Now, combine apple, cucumber, beans, turnip greens, and ginger in a juicer and process until juiced. Transfer to a serving glass and add few ice cubes.

Serve immediately.

Nutrition information per serving: Kcal: 122, Protein: 3.7g, Carbs: 34.2g, Fats: 0.8g

13. Ginger Pineapple Juice

Ingredients:

1 cup of pineapple, chunked

1 cup of watermelon, diced

2 cups of Iceberg lettuce, torn

¼ tsp of ginger, ground

Preparation:

Cut the top of the pineapple and peel it using a sharp paring knife. Peel it all and cut into small pieces. Fill the measuring cup and set aside.

Cut the top of the watermelon. Cut lengthwise in half and then cut one large wedge. Peel it and cut into small cubes. Remove the seeds and fill the measuring cup. Wrap the rest in a plastic foil and refrigerate for later.

Wash the lettuce thoroughly under cold running water. Drain and torn with your hands into small pieces. Set aside.

Now, combine pineapple, watermelon, and lettuce in a juicer and process until juiced. Transfer to a serving glass and stir in the ginger.

Serve immediately and enjoy!

Nutrition information per serving: Kcal: 127, Protein: 3.1g, Carbs: 35.8g, Fats: 0.6g

14.   Cinnamon Fuji Juice

Ingredients:

1 small Fuji apple, core and chopped

¼ tsp of cinnamon, ground

1 cup strawberries, chopped

1 cup of watermelon, diced

1 cup of fresh mint, torn

Preparation:

Wash the apple and cut in half. Remove the core and cut into bite-sized pieces. Set aside.

Wash the strawberries and remove the stems. Cut into bite-sized pieces and set aside.

Cut the top of the watermelon. Cut lengthwise in half and then cut one large wedge. Peel the wedge and cut into small cubes. Remove the seeds and fill the measuring cup. Wrap the rest in a plastic foil and refrigerate.

Wash the mint thoroughly and slightly drain. Torn with hands and set aside.

Now, combine apple, strawberries, watermelon, and mint

in a juicer and process until juiced. Transfer to a serving glass and stir in the cinnamon.

Add some crushed ice and serve immediately.

Nutrition information per serving: Kcal: 154, Protein: 3.5g, Carbs: 45.8g, Fats: 1.1g

15.   Watercress Cucumber Juice

Ingredients:

1 cup of watercress, chopped

1 cup of cucumber, sliced

1 small zucchini, chopped

1 cup of parsnip, sliced

1 oz water

Preparation:

Wash the watercress thoroughly under cold running water. Drain and chop into small pieces. Set aside.

Wash the cucumber and cut into thin slices. Fill the measuring cup and reserve the rest for later. Set aside.

Peel the zucchini and cut into thin slices. Set aside.

Wash the parsnip and trim off the green parts. slightly peel and cut into slices. Set side.

Now, combine watercress, cucumber, zucchini, and parsnip in a juicer and process until juiced. Transfer to a serving glass and stir in the water.

Add some ice and serve immediately.

Nutrition information per serving: Kcal: 99, Protein: 4.2g, Carbs: 29.9g, Fats: 0.9g

16.   Lettuce Asparagus Juice

Ingredients:

2 cups of Romaine lettuce, shredded

1 cup of asparagus, trimmed

5 large radishes, chopped

2 whole leeks, chopped

2 cups of cucumber, sliced

Preparation:

Wash the lettuce thoroughly under cold running water. Shred it and fill the measuring cups. Reserve the rest for later.

Wash the asparagus and trim off the woody ends. Cut into bite-sized pieces and set aside.

Wash the radishes and trim off the green parts. slightly peel and cut into thin slices. Set aside.

Wash the leeks and cut into bite-sized pieces. Set aside.

Wash the cucumber and cut into thin slices. Fill the measuring cups and reserve the rest in the refrigerator.

Now, combine lettuce, asparagus, radishes, leeks, and

cucumber in a juicer and process until juiced. Transfer to a serving glass and add some crushed ice before serving.

Enjoy!

Nutrition information per serving: Kcal: 137, Protein: 7.3g, Carbs: 37g, Fats: 1g

17.   Avocado Apple Juice

Ingredients:

1 cup of avocado, cubed

1 small Red Delicious apple, cored

1 cup of fresh basil, chopped

1 small peach, chopped

1 oz of milk

Preparation:

Peel the avocado and cut in half. Remove the pit and cut into small cubes. Fill the measuring cup and reserve the rest for later.

Wash the apple and cut lengthwise in half. Remove the core and cut into bite-sized pieces. Set aside.

Wash the basil thoroughly under cold running water. Slightly drain and chop into small pieces. Set aside.

Wash the peach and cut in half. Remove the pit and chop into small pieces. Set aside.

Now, combine basil, avocado, apple, and peach in a juicer and process until well juiced. Transfer to a serving glass and stir in the milk.

Add some ice and serve immediately.

Enjoy!

Nutrition information per serving: Kcal: 317, Protein: 6.5g, Carbs: 46.7g, Fats: 23.8g

18.   Banana Raspberry Juice

Ingredients:

1 medium-sized banana, sliced

1 cup of raspberries

2 medium-sized pears, chopped

1 cup of cucumber, sliced

Preparation:

Peel the banana and cut into small chunks. Set aside.

Wash the raspberries using a colander. Slightly drain and set aside.

Wash the pear and cut in half. Remove the core and cut into bite-sized pieces. Set aside.

Wash the cucumber and cut into thin slices. Fill the measuring cup and reserve the rest for later.

Now, combine banana, raspberries, pear, and cucumber in a juicer and process until juiced. Transfer to a serving glass and serve.

Enjoy!

Nutrition information per serving: Kcal: 290, Protein: 4.4g, Carbs: 97.7g, Fats: 1.8g

19.   Celery Apple Juice

Ingredients:

1 large celery stalk, chopped

1 small Fuji apple, cored

1 tbsp of aloe juice

1 cup of cucumber, sliced

1 medium-sized banana, sliced

Preparation:

Wash the celery stalk and chop into bite-sized pieces. Set aside.

Wash the apple and cut in half. Remove the core and cut into bite-sized pieces. Set aside.

Wash the cucumber and cut into thin slices. Fill the measuring cup and reserve the rest for later. Set aside.

Peel the banana and cut into chunks. Set aside.

Now, combine celery apple, cucumber, and banana in a juicer. Process until juiced.

Transfer to a serving glass and stir in the aloe juice.

Add some crushed ice and serve immediately.

Nutrition information per serving: Kcal: 174, Protein: 2.7g, Carbs: 50.3g, Fats: 0.8g

20. Ginger Lettuce Juice

Ingredients:

1 cup of Romaine lettuce, torn

¼ tsp of ginger, ground

1 cup of pineapple, chunked

1 cup of fresh mint, torn

1 cup of watercress, chopped

Preparation:

Combine lettuce, watercress, and mint in a large colander. Wash thoroughly under cold running water and torn into small pieces. Set aside.

Cut the top of the pineapple and peel it using a sharp paring knife. Peel it and cut into small pieces. Set aside.

Now, combine lettuce, pineapple, mint, and watercress in a juicer. Process until juiced.

Transfer to a serving glass and add some ice before serving.

Enjoy!

Nutrition information per serving: Kcal: 90, Protein: 3.2g, Carbs: 27.3g, Fats: 0.6g

21.   Fuji Chia Juice

Ingredients:

2 large Fuji apples, cored

1 tbsp of chia seeds

3 large carrots, sliced

½ tsp of ginger, ground

Preparation:

Core the apples and chop into bite-sized pieces. Combine with carrots.

Soak chia seeds in 4 tablespoons of hot water for 10 minutes.

Wash the carrots and chop into small pieces. Place them in a small bowl and set aside.

Now, process apples, chia, carrots, and in a juicer until well juiced. Transfer to serving glasses and stir in the chia seeds.

Refrigerate for 10 minutes before serving.

Enjoy!

Nutrition information per serving: Kcal: 177, Protein: 3.2g, Carbs: 28.4g, Fats: 4.6g

22.   Pineapple Lemon Juice

Ingredients:

1 cup of pineapple, peeled and chopped

½ large lemon, peeled

1 cup of watermelon, peeled and seeded

½ tsp of ginger, ground

1 oz milk

Preparation:

Using a sharp paring knife, peel and the pineapple. Chop into bite-sized pieces and fill the measuring cup. Reserve the rest for later.

Peel the lemon and cut in half. Set aside.

Peel and chop the watermelon. Remove the seeds. Set aside.

Now, process pineapple, lemon, and watermelon in a juicer. Transfer to serving glasses and stir in the ginger and milk.

Add some ice and serve immediately.

Nutrition information per serving: Kcal: 45, Protein: 2.3g, Carbs: 11.3g, Fats: 1.4g

23.   Spinach Parsley Juice

Ingredients:

½ cup of fresh spinach, torn

2 tbsp of fresh parsley, torn

2 large carrots, sliced

2 large apples, cored

¼ tsp of ginger, ground

1 tbsp of flaxseed

Preparation:

Rinse the spinach and parsley using a large colander. Drain and torn with your hands and set aside.

Chop the carrots into small pieces and place them in a bowl.

Wash and core the apples. Cut into bite-sized pieces and set aside.

Now, process spinach, parsley, carrots, and apples until well juiced. Transfer to serving glasses and stir in the ginger. Sprinkle with some flaxseeds and serve immediately!

Nutrition information per serving: Kcal: 119, Protein: 4.3g, Carbs: 62.2g, Fats: 2.3g

24.   Orange Carrot Juice

Ingredients:

2 large oranges, peeled

1 large cucumber, peeled

1 large carrot, sliced

1 cup of broccoli, chopped

Preparation:

Peel the oranges and cut into wedges.

Wash the carrot and slighlty peel. Cut into thin slices and set aside.

Peel the cucumber and cut into bite-sized pieces and aside.

Wash the broccoli thoroughly. Cut into bite-sized pieces and set aside.

Now, process oranges, carrot, cucumber, and broccoli in a juicer until juiced. Transfer to a serving glass and, optionally, stir in some honey or maple syrup.

Stir well with a spoon and add some ice cubes before serving.

Nutrition information per serving: Kcal: 68, Protein: 2.3g, Carbs: 19.7g, Fats: 0.1g

25.   Lime Pear Juice

Ingredients:

1 lime, peeled

1 large pear, cored

1 cup of green grapes

2 large cucumbers

Preparation:

Peel the lime and cut into quarters. Set aside.

Wash the pear and remove the core. Cut into bite-sized pieces and set aside.

Wash the green grapes under cold running water and drain using colander. Set aside.

Noe, process, lime, pear, grapes, and cucumbers in a juicer. Process until juiced. Transfer to serving glasses and stir well.

Refrigerate for 25 minutes before serving.

Enjoy!

Nutrition information per serving: Kcal: 113, Protein: 18.3g, Carbs: 31.3g, Fats: 0.1g

26.   Orange Celery Juice

Ingredients:

1 large orange, peeled

1 cup celery, chopped

6 medium-sized radishes, chopped

1 small fennel, chopped

1 whole cucumber, sliced

Preparation:

Peel the orange and divide into wedges.

Wash the celery and roughly chop into pieces. Set aside.

Wash and cut the radishes into small pieces. Set aside.

Trim off the fennel stalks and wilted outer layers. Wash and cut into bite-sized pieces and set aside.

Wash the cucumber and chop into small pieces.

Process orange, celery, radishes, fennel and cucumber in a juicer. Transfer to serving glasses and add some water to adjust the thickness, if needed.

Add some ice and serve.

Nutrition information per serving: Kcal: 110, Protein: 6.1g, Carbs: 28.7g, Fats: 1.2g

27.   Lemon Rosemary Juice

Ingredients:

2 whole lemon, peeled

½ tsp of fresh rosemary

3 whole grapefruits, peeled

2 large oranges, peeled

Preparation:

Peel the lemon and cut into quarters. Set aside.

Peel grapefruits and divide into wedges. Cut each wedge in half and set aside.

Peel the oranges and divide into wedges. Set aside.

Now, process grapefruits and oranges. Transfer to serving glasses and sprinkle with fresh rosemary for some extra flavor.

If you don't like rosemary, you can replace it with fresh mint.

Enjoy!

Nutrition information per serving: Kcal: 137, Protein: 3.2g, Carbs: 35.5g, Fats: 0.1g

28.   Sweet Pomegranate Juice

Ingredients:

½ cup of pomegranate seeds

½ cup of fresh kale

1 large Golden Delicious apple, cored

¼ tsp of ginger, ground

1 tbsp maple syrup

Preparation:

Cut the top of the pomegranate fruit using a sharp knife. slice down to each of the white membranes inside of the fruit. Pop the seeds into a medium sized bowl.

Wash thoroughly the kale. Drain and roughly chop it. Set aside.

Wash the apple and remove the core. Cut into bite-sized pieces and set aside.

Process the pomegranate seeds, kale, and apple in a juicer until well juiced.

Transfer to serving glasses and stir in the ginger. Add some water to adjust the thickness and stir in the maple syrup.

Optionally, garnish with mint leaves.

Add few ice cubes and serve immediately.

Nutrition information per serving: Kcal: 194, Protein: 6.2g, Carbs: 54.2g, Fats: 2.4g

29.   Lemon Watercress Juice

Ingredients:

1 large lemon, peeled

1 cup of watercress, torn

1 cup of pineapple, chunked

2 large carrots, sliced

2 tsp of fresh ginger, grated

Preparation:

Peel the lemon and cut into quarters. Set aside.

Wash the watercress and carrots. Torn the watercress with your hands and set aside. Using a sharp paring knife, carefully slice carrots into thin slices. Set aside.

Peel the pineapple and cut into small chunks. Set aside.

Peel the ginger root slice and cut into halves.

Process lemon, watercress, pineapple, carrots and ginger. Transfer to serving glasses and add a little bit of water or milk to adjust the thickness of the juice.

Add some ice and serve.

Nutrition information per serving: Kcal: 101, Protein: 3.1g, Carbs: 34.2g, Fats: 1.1g

30.   Chia Pepper Juice

Ingredients:

1 large yellow bell pepper, seeded

3 tbsp of chia seeds

1 large Golden Delicious apple, cored

1 whole lemon, peeled

Preparation:

Wash the bell pepper and cut into halves. Remove the seeds and then chop into small pieces.

Wash the apple and remove the core. Cut into bite-sized pieces and set aside.

Peel the lemon and cut into quarters. Set aside.

Process bell pepper, apple, and lemon in a juicer until juiced.

Transfer to serving glasses and stir in the chia seeds. Add a little bit of milk because chia will soak up the liquid.

Stir well and refrigerate for about 10 minutes before serving.

Enjoy!

Nutrition information per serving: Kcal: 135, Protein: 4.2g, Carbs: 31.3g, Fats: 6.2g

31.   Tomato Carrot Juice

Ingredients:

3 large tomatoes, chopped

4 large carrots,sliced

2 medium-sized zucchinis, peeled and chopped

1 cup asparagus, trimmed and chopped

Preparation:

Wash the tomatoes and cut into quarters. Cut in a bowl to reserve the juices. Set aside.

Wash the carrots and cut into small pieces. Set aside.

Peel the zucchinis and remove the seeds. Cut into bite-sized chunks and set aside.

Wash the asparagus and remove the woody ends. Chop into small pieces and set aside.

Combine tomatoes, carrots, zucchinis, and asparagus in a juicer and process until juiced.

Transfer to serving glasses and add a little bit of milk to adjust the thickness of the juice.

Serve immediately.

Nutrition information per serving: Kcal: 92, Protein: 5.4g, Carbs: 27.3g, Fats: 0.9g

32. Celery Mint Juice

Ingredients:

1 cup celery, chopped

¼ cup of fresh mint

1 large lime, peeled

3 oz of coconut water

¼ cup of fresh spinach

Preparation:

Wash the celery stalks and chop into small pieces. Set aside.

Wash the spinach and mint in a colander. Chop and place in a medium bowl. Add lukewarm water and let it stand for 5 minutes.

Peel the lime and cut into quarters. Set aside.

Now, combine celery, mint, lime, and spinach in a juicer and process until juiced.

Transfer to serving glasses and stir in the coconut water.

Refrigerate for 10 minutes and serve!

Nutrition information per serving: Kcal: 45, Protein: 2.2g, Carbs: 16.8g, Fats: 1.6g

33.   Carrot Lemon Juice

Ingredients:

3 large carrots

1 large lemon, peeled

1 medium-sized cucumber

1 large pear, cored

¼ cup of fresh mint

½ cup of broccoli

1 small ginger root slice, 1-inch

½ tsp of green tea powder

Preparation:

Wash the carrots and cut into small pieces. Set aside.

Peel the lemon and cut into quarters. Set aside.

Wash and cut the cucumber into small pieces. Set aside.

Wash the pear and remove the core. Cut into bite-sized pieces and set aside.

Combine broccoli and mint in a colander and wash under cold running water. Drain and set aside.

Peel the ginger root and set aside.

Combine tea powder and hot water in a small cup. Let it stand for 10 minutes.

Now, combine carrots, lemon, cucumber, pear, mint, broccoli, and ginger in a juicer. Process until nicely juiced.

Transfer to serving glasses and stir in the tea powder mixture.

Add some ice and serve!

Nutrition information per serving: Kcal: 141, Protein: 5.5g, Carbs: 45.7g, Fats: 0.9g

34.   Sweet Grapefruit Juice

Ingredients:

1 cup of grapefruit, chopped

1 tsp of liquid honey

2 large oranges, peeled

¼ tsp of ginger, ground

Preparation:

Peel the grapefruit and divide into wedges.. Cut each wedge in half and set aside.

Peel the oranges and divide into wedges. Set aside.

Wash the kale leaves and roughly chop it.

Now, process grapefruit and oranges in a juicer. Transfer to serving glasses and add some water to adjust the thickness if needed. Stir in the liquid honey and ginger.

Add some ice and serve immediately.

Nutrition information per serving: Kcal: 128, Protein: 7.3g, Carbs: 34.5g, Fats: 1.1g

35.   Carrot Orange Juice

Ingredients:

2 large carrots

1 large orange, peeled

1 cup of fresh strawberries

2 large Fuji apples, cored

1 large bell pepper, seeded

Preparation:

Wash carrots and cut into small pieces. Set aside.

Peel the orange and divide into wedges. Set aside.

Wash strawberries and cut them into halves. Set aside.

Wash apples and cut in half. Remove the core and cut into bite-sized pieces. Set aside.

Wash the bell pepper and cut into halves. Remove the seeds and cut into small pieces.

Now, process carrots, orange, strawberries, apples and bell pepper in a juicer. Transfer to the serving glasses and stir in the reserved tomato juice.

Refrigerate for 15 minutes before serving.

Nutrition information per serving: Kcal: 104, Protein: 3.9g, Carbs: 31.2g, Fats: 1.1g

36.   Swiss Chard Ginger Juice

Ingredients:

1 cup of Swiss chard, torn

¼ tsp of ginger, ground

1 tsp of green tea powder

2 cups of spinach, torn

1 cup of watercress, torn

1 cup of kale, torn

1 oz of water

Preparation:

Combine Swiss chard, spinach, watercress, and kale in a large colander. Wash thoroughly under cold running water. Slightly drain and torn into small pieces.

Place the tea powder in a small bowl. Add 3 tbsp of hot water and stir well. Set aside for 3 minutes.

Now, combine Swiss chard, spinach, watercress, and kale in a juicer and process until juiced. Transfer to a serving glass and stir in the ginger and water.

Refrigerate for 10 minutes before serving.

Enjoy!

Nutrition information per serving: Kcal: 87, Protein: 16.3g, Carbs: 22.9g, Fats: 2.4g

37.   Cinnamon Papaya Juice

Ingredients:

1 cup of papaya, chopped

¼ tsp of cinnamon, ground

1 whole grapefruit, peeled

1 large orange, peeled

1 cup of cucumber, sliced

2 tbsp of coconut water

Preparation:

Peel the papaya and cut into small chunks. Fill the measuring cup and reserve the rest in the refrigerator.

Peel the grapefruit and orange. Divide into wedges. Cut each wedge in half and set aside.

Wash the cucumber and cut into thin slices. Fill the measuring cup and reserve the rest for later.

Now, combine papaya, grapefruit, orange, and cucumber in a juicer and process until well juiced.

Transfer to a serving glass and stir in the cinnamon and coconut water.

Refrigerate for 5 minutes before serving.

Nutrition information per serving: Kcal: 214, Protein: 4.6g, Carbs: 65.4g, Fats: 1g

38.   Avocado Turmeric Juice

Ingredients:

1 cup of avocado, cubed

¼ tsp of turmeric, ground

1 cup of artichoke, chopped

1 cup of fresh spinach, torn

1 cup of green cabbage, torn

Preparation:

Trim off the outer layers of the artichoke using a sharp paring knife. Cut into bite-sized pieces and fill the measuring cup. Reserve the rest for later.

Combine spinach and cabbage in a large colander. Wash thoroughly under cold running water. Drain and torn into small pieces. Set aside.

Peel the avocado and cut lengthwise in half. Remove the pit and cut into small cubes. Fill the measuring cup and reserve the rest in the refrigerator.

Now, combine avocado, artichoke, spinach, and cabbage in a juicer and process until juiced. Transfer to a serving glass and stir in the turmeric.

Refrigerate for 5 minutes before serving.

Nutrition information per serving: Kcal: 282, Protein: 15.4g, Carbs: 42.6g, Fats: 23.2g

39.   Grapefruit Apple Juice

Ingredients:

1 whole grapefruit, peeled and wedged

1 small Red Delicious apple, cored

2 whole lemons, peeled and halved

1 cup of mango, chunked

¼ tsp of ginger, ground

1 tbsp agave nectar

1 oz of milk

Preparation:

Peel the grapefruit and divide into wedges. Cut each wedge in half and set aside.

Wash the apple and cut lengthwise in half. Remove the core and cut into bite-sized pieces. Set aside.

Peel the lemons and cut each lengthwise in half. Set aside.

Peel the mango and cut into chunks. Fill the measuring cup and reserve the rest for later. Set aside.

Now, combine grapefruit, apple emon, and mango in a

juicer and process until juiced. Transfer to serving glasses and stir in the ginger, milk, and agave.

Add few ice cubes and serve immediately.

Enjoy!

Nutrition information per serving: Kcal: 155, Protein: 4.5g, Carbs: 23.8g, Fats: 1.8g

40. Cinnamon Watermelon Juice

Ingredients:

1 cup of watermelon, chunked

¼ tsp of cinnamon, ground

1 large pear, chopped

1 cup of cranberries

1 whole lemon, peeled

1 oz of water

Preparation:

Cut the watermelon in half. Cut one large wedge and wrap the rest in a plastic foil and refrigerate. Peel the slice and cut into small cubes. Remove the pits and fill the measuring cup. Set aside.

Wash the pear and cut in half. Remove the core and cut into small pieces. Set aside.

Place the cranberries in a colander and rinse under cold running water. Drain and set aside.

Peel the lemon and cut lengthwise in half. Set aside.

Now, combine watermelon, pear, cranberries, and lemon

in a juicer and process until well juiced. Transfer to a serving glass and stir in the cinnamon and water.

Refrigerate for 15 minutes before serving.

Nutrition information per serving: Kcal: 186, Protein: 2.8g, Carbs: 64.1g, Fats: 0.8g

41. Spicy Cantaloupe Mint Juice

Ingredients:

1 cup of cantaloupe, chopped

1 cup of fresh mint, torn

1 large orange, peeled

1 whole plum, chopped

¼ tsp of turmeric, ground

¼ tsp of ginger, ground

Preparation:

Cut the cantaloupe in half. Scoop out the seeds and flesh. Cut and peel one large wedge. Chop into chunks and fill the measuring cup. Reserve the rest of the cantaloupe in a refrigerator.

Wash the mint thoroughly under cold running water. Torn into small pieces and set aside.

Peel the orange and divide into wedges. Cut each wedge in half and set aside.

Wash the plum and cut in half. Remove the pit and chop into small pieces. Set aside.

Now, combine cantaloupe, mint, orange, and plum in a juicer and process until juiced. Transfer to a serving glass and stir in the turmeric and ginger.

Add some ice and serve immediately.

Enjoy!

Nutrition information per serving: Kcal: 151, Protein: 4.4g, Carbs: 45.6g, Fats: 0.9g

42.   Pepper Rosemary Juice

Ingredients:

1 large green bell pepper, chopped

1 tsp of rosemary, finely chopped

1 medium-sized tomato, chopped

1 cup of fresh spinach, torn

1 whole lemon, peeled

Preparation:

Wash the bell pepper and cut in half. Remove the stem and seeds. Cut into small pieces and set aside.

Wash the tomato and place in a small bowl. Chop into small pieces and reserve the tomato juice while cutting. Set aside.

Wash the spinach thoroughly under cold running water. Drain and torn into small pieces. Set aside.

Peel the lemon and cut lengthwise in half. Set aside.

Now, combine bell pepper, tomato, spinach, and lemon in a juicer and process until juiced. Transfer to a serving glass and stir in the rosemary.

Add few ice cubes and serve immediately.

Nutrition information per serving: Kcal: 92, Protein: 9.3g, Carbs: 27.7g, Fats: 1.7g

43.　Apple Lime Juice

Ingredients:

1 small Golden Delicious apple, cored

1 whole lime, peeled

¼ tsp of cinnamon, ground

1 cup of watermelon, chopped

1 large banana, chopped

1 cup of fresh mint, torn

Preparation:

Wash the apple and cut lengthwise in half. Remove the core and chop into bite-sized pieces. Set aside.

Peel the lime and cut lengthwise in half. Set aside.

Wash the mint thoroughly under cold running water. Drain and torn into small pieces. Set aside.

Cut the watermelon in half. Cut one large wedge and wrap the rest in a plastic foil and refrigerate. Peel the slice and cut into small cubes. Remove the pits and fill the measuring cup. Set aside.

Peel the banana and cut into small chunks. Set asid

Now, combine apple, lime, watermelon, banana, and mint in a juicer and process until juiced. Transfer to a serving glass and stir in the cinnamon.

Add some crushed ice and serve immediately.

Nutrition information per serving: Kcal: 239, Protein: 4.2g, Carbs: 69.5g, Fats: 1.2g

44.   Raspberry Ginger Juice

Ingredients:

1 cup of raspberries

¼ tsp of ginger, ground

1 cup of spinach, chopped

1 medium-sized wedge of honeydew melon

1 small Golden Delicious apple, cored

Preparation:

Place the raspberries in a colander and rinse well under cold running water. Drain and set aside.

Wash the spinach thoroughly under cold running water. Drain and chop into small pieces. Set aside.

Cut melon lengthwise in half. Scoop out the seeds and then wash the melon. Cut one wedge and peel it. Cut into bite-sized pieces and set aside. Reserve the rest in the refrigerator.

Wash the apple and cut lengthwise in half. Remove the core and cut into bite-sized pieces. Set aside.

Now, combine raspberries, spinach, melon, and apple in a

juicer and process until juiced. Transfer to a serving glass and stir in the ginger. Add some ice before serving.

Enjoy!

Nutrition information per serving: Kcal: 142, Protein: 4.5g, Carbs: 46.1g, Fats: 1.4g

45.   Coconut Blueberry Juice

Ingredients:

1 oz of coconut water

1 cup of blueberries

2 cups of raspberries

1 medium-sized zucchini, sliced

1 small ginger knob, peeled

Preparation:

Combine blueberries and raspberries in a large colander. Rinse well under cold running water. Drain and set aside.

Wash the zucchini and cut into thin slices. Set aside.

Peel the ginger knob and cut into small pieces. Set aside.

Now, combine blueberries, raspberries, zucchini, and ginger in a juicer and process until juiced. Transfer to a serving glass and stir in the coconut water.

Add crushed ice or refrigerate for 5 minutes before serving.

Enjoy!

Nutrition information per serving: Kcal: 164, Protein: 6.5g, Carbs: 58g, Fats: 2.7g

46.   Plum Apple Juice

Ingredients:

1 whole plum, chopped

1 medium-sized Fuji apple, cored

1 cup of mango, chopped

1 large peach, chopped

1 oz of coconut water

Preparation:

Wash the plum and cut in half. Remove the pit and chop into small pieces. Set aside.

Wash the apple cut lengthwise in half. Remove the core and chop into small pieces. Set aside.

Peel the mango and cut into small cubes. Fill the measuring cup and reserve the rest for later.

Wash the peach and cut lengthwise in half. Remove the pit and cut into small pieces. Set aside.

Now, combine plum, apple, mango, and peach in a juicer and process until juiced. Transfer to a serving glass and stir in the coconut water.

Add some ice and serve immediately.

Nutrition information per serving: Kcal: 252, Protein: 3.8g, Carbs: 71.1g, Fats: 1.6g

47.　　Lime Apple Juice

Ingredients:

1 whole lime, peeled

1 small Granny Smith's apple, cored

1 cup of pomegranate seeds

1 cup of blueberries

¼ tsp of ginger, ground

2 oz of water

Preparation:

Peel the lime and cut lengthwise in half. Set aside.

Wash the apple and cut lengthwise in half. Remove the core and cut into bite-sized pieces and set aside.

Cut the top of the pomegranate fruit using a sharp paring knife. Slice down to each of the white membranes inside of the fruit. Pop the seeds into a measuring cup and set aside.

Place the blueberries in a colander. Rinse well under cold running water and drain. Set aside.

Now, combine lime, apple, pomegranate seeds, blueberries in a juicer and process until juiced. Transfer to a serving glass and stir in the ginger and water.

Refrigerate for 5 minutes before serving.

Enjoy!

Nutrition information per serving: Kcal: 206, Protein: 3.3g, Carbs: 61.1g, Fats: 1.8g

48.   Cucumber Zucchini Juice

Ingredients:

1 cup of cucumber, sliced

1 small zucchini, cubed

1 cup of fennel, sliced

1 large yellow bell pepper, chopped

1 cup of Romaine lettuce, chopped

Preparation:

Wash the cucumber and cut into thin slices. Fill the measuring cup and reserve the rest for later.

Wash the zucchini and cut into small cubes. Set aside.

Trim off the fennel bulb and remove the green parts. Wash it and cut into small pieces. Fill the measuring cup and reserve the rest for later. Set aside.

Wash the bell pepper and cut lengthwise in half. Remove the stem and seeds. Cut into small pieces and set aside.

Wash the Romaine lettuce thoroughly under cold running water. Drain and chop into small pieces. Set aside.

Now, combine cucumber, zucchini, fennel, bell pepper, and

lettuce in a juicer and process until juiced. Transfer to a serving glass and refrigerate for 5 minutes before serving.

Nutrition information per serving: Kcal: 85, Protein: 5.3g, Carbs: 25.2g, Fats: 1.1g

49.   Coconut Lime Juice

Ingredients:

2 oz of coconut water

1 whole lime, peeled and halved

1 large orange, peeled

1 cup of broccoli, chopped

1 cup of cucumber, sliced

¼ tsp of ginger, ground

Preparation:

Peel the lime and cut lengthwise in half. Set aside.

Peel the orange and divide into wedges. Cut each wedge in half and set aside.

Wash the broccoli and trim off the outer leaves. Cut into small pieces and fill the measuring cup. Reserve the rest in the refrigerator.

Wash the cucumber and cut into thin slices. Fill the measuring cup and reserve the rest for later.

Now, combine lime, orange, broccoli, and cucumber in a juicer and process until juiced. Transfer to a serving glass and stir in the coconut water and ginger. Add some ice and serve immediately.

Nutrition information per serving: Kcal: 106, Protein: 4.8g, Carbs: 33.3g, Fats: 0.6g

50. Lemon Apple Juice

Ingredients:

1 whole lemon, peeled

1 large Fuji apple, cored and chopped

2 large bananas, peeled and chopped

1 cup of fresh mint, torn

1 whole kiwi, peeled

¼ tsp of cinnamon, ground

Preparation:

Peel the lemon and cut lengthwise in half. Set aside.

Wash the apple and cut lengthwise in half. Remove the core and cut into bite-sized pieces. Set aside.

Peel the bananas and cut into small pieces. Set aside.

Wash the mint thoroughly under cold running water. Drain and torn into small pieces. Set aside.

Now, combine lemon, apple, bananas, mint, and kiwi in a juicer and process until well juiced. Transfer to a serving glass and stir in the cinnamon.

Add some ice and serve immediately.

Enjoy!

Nutrition information per serving: Kcal: 398, Protein: 6.1g, Carbs: 117g, Fats: 2.1g

51.   Pear Coconut Juice

Ingredients:

1 small pear, chopped

2 oz of coconut water

1 cup of avocado, cubed

2 whole plums, chopped

1 whole lime, pitted and chopped

¼ tsp of ginger, ground

Preparation:

Wash the pear and cut in half. Remove the core and into bite-sized pieces. Set side.

Peel the avocado and cut lengthwise in half. Remove the pit and cut into small cubes. Fill the measuring cup and reserve the rest for later.

Wash the plums and cut in half. Remove the pits and cut into small pieces. Set aside.

Peel the lime and cut lengthwise in half. Set aside.

Now, combine pear, avocado, plums, and lime in a juicer and process until juiced. Transfer to a serving glass and stir in the coconut water and ginger.

Add some ice and serve immediately.

Nutrition information per serving: Kcal: 328, Protein: 4.6g, Carbs: 54.1g, Fats: 22.6g

52.   Lemon Apple Juice

Ingredients:

1 whole lemon, peeled

1 small Fuji apple, cored

1 cup of blueberries

1 cup of cherries, pitted

1 large banana, peeled

¼ tsp of cinnamon, ground

Preparation:

Peel the lemon and cut lengthwise in half. Set aside.

Wash the apple and cut lengthwise in half. Remove the core and cut into small pieces. Set aside.

Rinse the blueberries using a large colander. Drain and set aside.

Wash the cherries and cut in half. Remove the pits and stems. Set aside.

Peel the banana and cut into small chunks. Set aside.

Now, combine lemon, apple, blueberries, cherries, and

banana in a juicer and process until juiced. Transfer to a serving glass and stir in the cinnamon.

Add some ice and serve immediately.

Nutrition information per serving: Kcal: 340, Protein: 5.5g, Carbs: 98.1g, Fats: 1.7g

53. Banana Zucchini Juice

Ingredients:

1 large banana, chopped

1 medium-sized zucchini, sliced

1 large Golden Delicious apple, cored

1 large orange, peeled and wedged

2 oz of water

Preparation:

Peel the banana and cut into small chunks. Set aside.

Peel the zucchini and cut in half. Scoop out the seeds and cut into small pieces. Set aside.

Wash the apple and remove the core. Cut into bite-sized pieces and set aside.

Peel the orange and divide into wedges. Set aside.

Now, process banana, zucchini, apple, and orange in a juicer.

Transfer to serving glasses and refrigerate for 10 minutes before serving.

Enjoy!

Nutrition information per serving: Kcal: 296, Protein: 6.5g, Carbs: 86.8g, Fats: 1.7g

54.   Zucchini Broccoli Juice

Ingredients:

1 cup of leeks, chopped

1 cup of fresh parsley, torn

1 large zucchini

1 cup of broccoli, chopped

A handful of spinach, torn

2 oz of water

Preparation:

Wash the leeks and roughly chop them. Set aside.

Wash the parsley and spinach thoroughly and torn with hands. Set aside.

Peel the zucchini and cut in half. Scoop out the seeds and chop into small pieces. Set aside.

Wash the broccoli and chop into small pieces. Set aside.

Now, combine leeks, parsley, zucchini, broccoli, and spinach in a juicer and process until juiced.

Transfer to serving glasses and stir in the water. Add some

ice and serve immediately.

Enjoy!

Nutrition information per serving: Kcal: 225, Protein: 13.1g, Carbs: 58.7g, Fats: 2.7g

55. Apple Mint Juice

Ingredients:

1 large Granny Smith's apple, cored

1 cup of fresh mint, torn

1 cup of blackberries

1 large orange, wedged

1 tbsp honey

2 oz coconut water

Preparation:

Wash the apple and remove the core. Cut into bite-sized pieces and set aside.

Place the mint in a bowl and add one cup of lukewarm water. Let it soak for 15 minutes.

Place the blackberries in a colander and wash under cold running water. Drain and set aside.

Peel the orange and divide into wedges. Set aside.

Now, combine apple, mint, blackberries, and orange in a juicer and process until juiced.

Transfer to serving glasses and stir in the coconut water and honey. Add some ice and serve immediately.

Enjoy!

Nutrition information per serving: Kcal: 287, Protein: 5.3g, Carbs: 88.4g, Fats: 1.5g

56.   Cucumber Turmeric Juice

Ingredients:

1 large cucumber, sliced

¼ tsp of turmeric, ground

1 cup of cantaloupe, chopped

1 cup of butternut squash, chopped

2 large carrots, sliced

1 oz of water

Preparation:

Wash the cucumber and carrots and cut into thick slices. Set aside.

Cut the cantaloupe in half. Scoop out the seeds and flesh. Cut two medium wedges and peel them. Chop into chunks and set aside. Reserve the rest of the cantaloupe in a refrigerator for some other juice.

Peel the butternut squash and remove the seeds using a spoon. Cut into small cubes and reserve the rest of the squash for some other recipe. Wrap in a plastic foil and refrigerate.

Now, combine carrots, cucumber, cantaloupe, and squash in a juicer and process until juiced.

Transfer to serving glasses and stir in the turmeric and water.

Refrigerate for 5 minutes before serving.

Enjoy!

Nutrition information per serving: Kcal: 182, Protein: 6g, Carbs: 53.8g, Fats: 1.1g

57.   Sweet Apple Kale Juice

Ingredients:

1 large Fuji apple, cored

1 cup of fresh kale, torn

1 cup of strawberries, chopped

1 cup of cranberries

1 large cucumber, sliced

Preparation:

Wash the apple and remove the core. Cut into bite-sized pieces and set aside.

Wash the kale thoroughly and drain. Torn with hands and set aside.

Combine strawberries and cranberries in a colander and wash under cold running water. Drain and cut strawberries in half. Set aside.

Wash the cucumber and cut into thick slices. Set aside.

Now, process apple, kale, strawberries, cranberries, and cucumber. Transfer to serving glasses and add some ice cubes before serving.

Enjoy!

Nutrition information per serving: Kcal: 229, Protein: 7.4g, Carbs: 72g, Fats: 1.9g

58.   Avocado Vanilla Juice

Ingredients:

1 cup of avocado, chunked

¼ tsp of vanilla extract

1 large cucumber, sliced

1 cup of fresh mint, torn

3 whole kiwis, peeled

3 oz of water

Preparation:

Peel the avocado and cut in half. Remove the pit and cut into chunks. Reserve the rest for some other juice. Set aside.

Wash the cucumber and cut into thick slices. Set aside.

Wash the mint thoroughly under cold running water. Set aside.

Peel the kiwis and cut lengthwise in half. Set aside.

Now, combine avocado, cucumber, mint, and kiwis in a juicer and process until juiced. Transfer to serving glasses and stir in the water and vanilla extract.

Add some ice and serve immediately.

Enjoy!

Nutrition information per serving: Kcal: 351, Protein: 8.3g, Carbs: 57.8g, Fats: 23.6g

ADDITIONAL TITLES FROM THIS AUTHOR

70 Effective Meal Recipes to Prevent and Solve Being Overweight: Burn Fat Fast by Using Proper Dieting and Smart Nutrition

By

Joe Correa CSN

48 Acne Solving Meal Recipes: The Fast and Natural Path to Fixing Your Acne Problems in Less Than 10 Days!

By

Joe Correa CSN

41 Alzheimer's Preventing Meal Recipes: Reduce or Eliminate Your Alzheimer's Condition in 30 Days or Less!

By

Joe Correa CSN

70 Effective Breast Cancer Meal Recipes: Prevent and Fight Breast Cancer with Smart Nutrition and Powerful Foods

By

Joe Correa CSN

www.ingramcontent.com/pod-product-compliance
Lightning Source LLC
Chambersburg PA
CBHW030247030426
42336CB00009B/289